# Unlocking the truth:
## Day to day meal plan for maximum weight loss

Noel Johnson

I0413961

## Why I wrote this book

I know personally what it means to be overweight "Heck" I use to be overweight myself...

## Why should you read this book?

This book will help you lose weight

# Copyright

# Table of Contents

# Introduction

This book was design to be informative, easy to understand and easily approachable. We want you to understand the reasons for weight gain and why weight loss can be challenging and the meals you can take for weight loss.

If you have tried other weight loss guide and you have not gain the desired results, you might not feel confident and enthusiastic, you may even give up, well I am here to tell you that don't give up.

What these other programs leave out is the mindset, the will power, and a meticulous meal plan that you should follow day by day. It's very important to realize that what you eat today determines what you look like tomorrow. You must be willing to sacrifice your old ways and move into new habits. This program will not only transform you physically it will also transform you mentally.

I'm sure many of you are skeptical about this program and probably asking yourself, "Does this program really work?" keep reading to find out.

Once the information is obtained and understood your next step is to put it in "action". This is a scientifically proven meal plan, that is design for maximizing weight loss efficiency.

# Innovation of weight loss

There are many weight programs out there that claim they can help you with weight loss, but always turn out in disappointment. I know this because I use to by a victim myself, the internet is scattered with abundance of information aiming to extract low wage earners money from people like ourselves. I am here to change that, I am giving you guys information that will change the way you approach your daily meals. One of the success behind this weight loss program is that it breaks down your day to day meal plan, by giving you a detailed healthy food plan that you should take three time throughout each day. Unlike other weight loss programs, my program is design to give you the result you desire during the first week of applying it. There has never been a diet this in depth that will not only give you specific meals, but explain the psychology of each meal plan. Because of our in-depth analysis, customers from all over the world are reporting massive breakthrough in their life and are beginning to see massive results. This diet is different from other meal plan that involve supplement, rather it focuses on healthy food that is scientifically proven and result oriented. Result is what this program strives to achieve, I will not be satisfied until you are satisfied.

This program will focus more on what you eat and how your mind can be your worse enemy if it is not controlled. The meal plan is very simple to follow, but considering the nature of outside forces such as controlling your mindset, being discipline, and worshiping old habits. These three elements can be difficult to maneuver and the better you can control each the more result you will gain. Old habits die hard, most of you might disagree, but the truth is, this applies to you one way or another. It very hard to give up something that you have been doing for a long time, it takes practice and practice become permanent.

The information presented in this book is backed by research, it is not like other book that is filled with empty promises. It is designed out of years of research and proven results tailored for anyone looking to lose weight. This meal plan is tried and have already given millions of people the body that they never imagine was possible.

Millions of people around the world commit themselves to yoga classes, hard diets, and intense exercises. We receive thousands of complained each year, they also asked question like why are they not losing weight?

We often have four answers

1) Your mindset need to be focus

2) Your meal plan is not meticulously designed

3) You need to be fully committed

4) Your meal plan need more nutrients dense food

# Weight loss begin with nutrients that is "backed" and "proven"

What you eat for breakfast, lunch and dinner can seriously impact your weight. Frosted flakes with added sugar, lunch packed with grease, to dinner filled with more added fat won't give you the outcome you want.

Committing to a healthy diet all too quickly can be difficult for some people. So, i recommend taking small steps. Usually many of my customers would message me and say that they can't seem to change what they are used to eating. For such reason, small step is recommended. Diets likes the one I am providing takes time to adapt and people usually fail when they move all too quickly from one diet to another.

# Food is your worse enemy

Food is one of our best friends and yet it's one of our worse enemies. It's quite sad to say that the one thing that should be keeping us alive is the one thing that is killing us. I wish some of what I just said were untrue, but it's the indisputable truth. We live in a society dominated by "food fanatics", people who consumed any and everything. Relying on the food you eat leave you vulnerable and that's why a change in lifestyle is inevitable. Our era is filled with food choices and this makes us catch diseases, gain weight and hinders the body from function accordingly. Many of us blame any and everything, but we never held ourselves accountable. Watching what you eat and researching products ingredients is what will separate you from a person who is overweight to a person who have cancer. There is no straightforward way to detach yourself from the food you eat each day and the food you choose to eat tomorrow. Just always remember that what you eat now and how your body respond to it will determine how you look tomorrow. If I had known this concept earlier in my life, I would have never been overweight years ago. One of the ugly truth about me is that I never held myself accountable, especially for eating burger king five time a day. yes, I needed to quit, but it was hard, it took me years to finally face the truth and it was not long after that I decided to change. Limiting what you eat will not only save you, it will decrease your calories intake, while reducing your body fat percentage. Limit and choosing the right amount of calories intake will determine how quick your body gain weight or lose weight.

One of my key to success for me over the years is that I am detail oriented. Details matters, which means the more precisely you can follow a meal plan the more you will be able to lose weight. Don't let your nasty habits come in the way. I am telling you guys, because I am a victim of my nasty habits. When I started, my meal plan years ago I was well motivated, yet stubborn. The truth is dirty habits is your worse enemy, but it can be overcome through will power and determination. The same feel will try and overpower you, but always remember where you want to be.

# The Mindset

Mindset will carry you a far way, without it, it's likely your craving will get the better of you. What I always recommend to customers is to keep their mindset in check. They can do this by surrounding themselves with expected goal in mind. This means keeping a picture of a role model in your room, phone, and kitchen, somewhere you can see it daily, what this will do is it will program your mind and put you in a constant state of focus. Each time you see this picture it will motivate you and push you in the right direction. Your mind is like a computer, if you can program it to be more precise and focus, it can change your life. Your mindset is also one of your worse enemies, because when it is not in the right place, it is very hard to change. You should always strive to control your mindset, since the more control you have the more success rate you will get. My mindset was one of my greatest enemies, because it was never in the right place. The truth is I never really wanted to lose weight until my friends and family started to tell me how "fat" am getting. This is a dilemma that people face often in their life, and it's something we can draw strength from. I draw strength from my peers, my surrounding and from my role models. This helps strengthen my mindset and push me to eat better over the years. I won't say it was easy, because it was not, but when you truly desire something your mindset is just a small burden to overcome. Fixing your mindset will not only help you lose excessive weight in this meal plan, it will help you become a more successful person in life. I cannot reiterate enough how important your mindset is and the benefits it had brought me. Your mindset will open a new world of possibilities, it will be one of your important qualities that will transform you into a new person. It will transcend you to think higher and move you into that phase of continuous development.

# Day 1 meal plan

## BREAKFAST

1 Cup Skim Milk

1 Orange, medium

1 Cup Cheerios

MORNING SNACK

1 Cup Cantaloupe Melon

## Lunch

Vietnamese-Style Beef & Noodle Broth

1 Whole-Wheat Pita Bread, small

1 Cup Skim Milk

1 Fudgsicle, no sugar added


## AFTERNOON SNACK

2 Tablespoons Prepared Hummus

3 Ounces Celery Sticks

1 bottle of water


## DINNER

1/2 Cup Cooked Brown Rice

Green & Yellow Beans with Wild Mushrooms

Roasted Cod with Warm Tomato-Olive-Caper Tapenade

1/2 Banana, small

1 bottle of water

# Supercharge your health and boost your system

This meal plan above represents nutrients taken from the various food chart such as protein, carbohydrates, and vitamin. Healthy eating is not about consuming any and everything it includes; consuming high quality proteins, carbohydrates, heart-healthy fats, vitamins, and minerals. The purpose of this table is to minimize processed and high fat foods that we eat every day. Eating in this manner will helps you maintain your everyday body functions. Eating what the table provide will also promotes optimal body weight, and will assist in disease prevention. The nutrients in the table provided above will support your day-to-day living, protect your cells from environmental damage and repair any cellular damage that might occur. As you can see there is a lot of protein provided in table above, it will rebuild your injured tissue and promotes a healthy immune system. Vitamins A, C, and E, is also in this diet, it will act as an antioxidant to protect your cells against toxins, and B vitamins will help you extract energy.

# Super Orange

Oranges are extremely high in vitamin C, it is vital for producing, maintaining, and repairing your ligaments, skin, tendons, cartilage, and blood vessels. Oranges are also high in vitamin B-1, with 1 cup containing nearly 15 percent of your RDA. This vitamin will help your body deal with stress by providing a boost to your immune system. Oranges are major source of vitamin B-9. Orange will also help reduce your risk of stroke by keeping concentrations of the amino acid at normal levels. Oranges are rich in antioxidants, which help to eliminate potentially cancer-causing free radicals from your body. Orange should be one of your best friends during this meal plan.

# Orange linkage to weight loss

One cup of oranges contains only 85 calories, making this fruit very dense in nutrients and very low in calories. The same serving also contains 4.3 grams of dietary fiber. People who eat more fiber tend to gain less weight and fat than those who eat only small portion of fiber. High fiber food help with weight loss by staying in your stomach longer, compared to normal food. High fiber food takes time to chew and usually absorb water in your stomach. In addition, they slow the emptying of your stomach to keep you full most of the day. So, for anyone who is always eating this is a game changer, it will not only make you not angry, it will make you feel full most of the time throughout the day. Each medium orange provides 3.1 grams of fiber, which is roughly 12 percent of the daily value. Filling up on foods like oranges which are low in energy density, will help you lose weight rapidly. By eating orange, you can eat a larger amount without going over your calorie limit. In turn, you are less likely to feel hungry in between occasional snacks and meal. I know this might sound too good to be true, for some of you, because I felt the same way. Finding out this wonderful news about orange not only help me to eat less through the day, it transforms everything I know about orange, it helps me reduce my calories intake

# Day 2 meal plan

**Breakfast**

1 Cup Skim Milk

1/2 Banana, small

1 Cup Bran Flakes Cereal

MORNING SNACK

1 Fruit & Nut Granola Bar

**Lunch**

Spicy Thai Shrimp Salad

2 Cups Romaine Lettuce, shredded

1 Whole-Wheat Pita Bread, small

Chocolate-Raspberry

**Dinner**

1 Cup Steamed Brussels Sprouts

Almond-Crusted Chicken Fingers

2/3 Cup Cooked Couscous

# Calories restriction

A new study suggests that healthy people can achieve several benefits from simply eating less calories. There was a new study that compared the diets of 215 adults over the course of 3 years, participants who restricted what they ate reported significantly better cognitive and psychological effects, compared to the group that eat whatever they like. The participants were men and women aged between 19 and 48 years old. From this sample, one group was assigned to reduce their calories by 24 percent, while the other group didn't have to alter their regular diet. If you're thinking you'd much prefer to be in the eat whatever you want group, consider this: two years later, the calorie restriction group reported improved tone and reduced anxiety, plus improved general health. What's more fascinating is that, after one year on the new eating plan, they reported enjoying better sleep quality. They also lost weight, dropping almost 14 percent of their body weight at the end of two years, with the calories restriction group sitting on 22.6 by the end of the study. But before you rush to reduce your own food consumption, bear in mind it's not easy to slash your calorie intake by 25 percent. On the contrary, it's considered to be a pretty big adjustment. Couple of years ago, after researching my calories intake i realizing that, I was consuming too much, it became clear to me that I had to reduce my intake. If I had not made that decision long ago I would have never been where I am today. The math's is very simple 1 pound of fat equals 3,500 calories, once you determine how much calories you need per days subtract 1000 calories per day to create a 7000 calories deficit per week to lose 2 pound. Eating 1000 fewer calories per day won't be applicable to some people, it is just not possible. Women for instance burn between 1,300 to 1,200 calories per day, so cutting 1000 calories is nutritionally impossible, and this could affect their metabolism astronomically. Most people consumed a daily calorie between 1,200 to 1,500, which is basically low, but essential for weight loss.

# Why eat lots of fruits

Fruit is rich in a type of sugar that the body is very good at assimilating, and which is great for nourishing your brain early in the day. Remember, your brain needs about 22% of the total energy you use up throughout the day, and glucose is an essential fuel for many of its most basic functions. So, fruit is a great food to get your body going in the morning, as well as one that is very easy to digest. Fruit is also rich in water, fiber, vitamins, and minerals, which will help you stay hydrated throughout the day and prevent constipation.

# Confronting the myths of banana

Banana are nutritious, low energy density food, which is good for dropping excessive pounds. I know many people believe banana is associate with weight gain, but it's the opposite. The key to eating banana and avoiding weight gain is to pace yourself. Therefore, ½ banana is recommend in day 2. A banana supplies the perfect number of calories for a snack, but also has enough calories to ruin a diet if you meet your daily calorie goal, and then randomly add the banana. While bananas provide a range of nutrients, they are excellent sources of potassium and vitamin B-6. Resistant starch and fiber that bananas contain not only support weight loss, but also aid in digestive health. Fiber plays a key role in weight loss because it slows digestion, which helps you feel full and keeps blood sugar balanced. The key to using banana for weight loss is to not eat too much, However, make sure you include a small portion in your diet each day.

# Day 3 meal plan

**Breakfast**

1 Whole-Wheat English Muffin

1 Cup Skim Milk

1/2 Cup Blueberries

1 Teaspoon Fat Free Cream Cheese

MORNING SNACK

1 Apple, small

**Lunch**

1 Cup Tossed Salad Mix

1 Tablespoon Fat Free Blue Cheese Salad Dressing

Spanish Tortilla

1/2 Cup Fresh Pineapple

1 Slice Reduced-Calorie Oatmeal Bran Bread

**DINNER**

Simple Sautéed Spinach

1 Cup Skim Milk

Shrimp with Mango & Basil

1/2 Cup Cooke

# Staying committed

A lot of people would usually contact me and say they are not losing enough weight. I would usually tell them that they need to follow the meal plan day by day, lunch by lunch and dinner by dinner. It should be a continuous effort to eat according to what each day show as much as possible. Commitment is one of the most fundamental principles of success. Commitments are powerful because they influence how you sound, how you feel, and how you act toward something. Making a commitment means that you try harder, you don't consider quitting and you don't look back. A meaningful commitment gives you a script for how to handle things when times get tough. And make no mistake, everyone wants to quit at one time in their life. Unfortunately, most people quit when they feel like quitting, which is why they rarely succeed at anything. After numerous attempt to lose weight over the years, I've learned that, one of the most distinguishing characteristics of success is perseverance and commitment. People often set personal improvement goals, but usually quit after few days. The key is to anticipate "quitting" is to make yourself a promise that the feeling of wanting to quit will not overpower you. One of thing I always recommend to my customers is to always keep the end goal in mind, think of what you want to look like in few months from now. Once you decide, it's imperative that you follow through. When I think of the importance of following through, I'm reminded of one of the world most influential motivational speaker Zig Ziglar, known for encouraging people all over the world. He stated that "commitment that moved us into action, and discipline enabled us to follow through." People give up too easy and that's their biggest problem. I have had numerous customer told me that it is quite hard to stick to the meal plan, but I always told them that if is truly worth pursuing, they should stay on that path. Think about successful people like Steve Job and Oprah for instances they all have one thing in common they never gave up and look where they are now.

Be willing to stand up to the challenges and always keep expectation in mind. This is because expectation usually become reality. What are you committed to achieving? How hard and how long have you been working at it? Did you set your expectations too high? You must identify specific reasons why something is not working and fix it. I used to go to the gym three days a week, but I still could not see any results like the other people working out in the gym and trust me this did not sit well with me. I was confused, because I was desperate to find answers to my problem. It took me almost five years to realize that it is not just about working out its about what you eat. If you eat right you can achieve rapids results in weeks, rather than months. After researching, analyzing sport journals and listening to experts. I realize a pattern and this lead me to design and develop my ultimate eating plan. After testing my methods for weeks, I started to see unbelievable result. The result amazed me so much that I decided to share it with the world. One of the reason I wanted to share my meal plan design is that I know firsthand what it means when you are overweight and desperately desire to lose weight, but everything you try fails.

# Day 4 meal plan

**Breakfast**

1 Cup Skim Milk

1/2 Cup Hot Oatmeal

1 Ounce Dried Fruit

1 Tablespoon Walnuts

MORNING SNACK

1 Kiwi

**Lunch**

1 Cup Tossed Salad Mix

Puerto Rican Fish

1 Tablespoon Low Calorie Caesar Salad Dressing

1 Slice Reduced-Calorie Oatmeal Bran Bread

1 Cup Honeydew Melon

**Dinner**

1/2 Cup Cooked Brown Rice

Maple-Glazed Chicken Breasts

Roasted Squash & Fennel with Thyme

1/2 Cup Mango

# Daily food choices and implication

The food you choose each day affect your health, how you feel today, tomorrow, and in the future. Good nutrition is an important part of leading a healthy lifestyle. A well design diet will help you to reach and maintain a healthy weight, reduce your risk of chronic diseases, and promote your overall health. Unhealthy eating habits have contributed to the obesity epidemic in the United States. One-third of U.S. adults are obese and approximately 16% of children and adolescents aged 3—18 years are obese.  A poor diet is associated with major health risks that can cause illness and even death. These include heart disease, high blood pressure, type 2 diabetes, and certain types of cancer. According to the American Cancer Society, processed meats, fried meats, and alcohol are associated with an increased risk for certain types of cancer. A healthy diet is associated with a lower incidence of depression, anxiety disorders and dysthymia than a typical Western diet high in sugar, processed foods, and alcohol.

By making smart food choices, you can help protect yourself from these health problems. The risk factors for adult chronic diseases, like hypertension and type 2 diabetes, are increasingly seen in younger ages, often a result of unhealthy eating habits and increased weight gain. The linkage between good nutrition and healthy weight, is too important to ignore. By taking steps to eat healthy, you'll be on your way to getting the nutrients your body needs to stay fit, active, and strong.

# Day 5 meal plan

**Breakfast**

1 Scrambled Eggs

1 Slice Reduced-Calorie Oatmeal Bran Bread

1/2 Cup Grapefruit

1 Cup Skim Milk

MORNING SNACK

6 Ounces Nonfat Vanilla or Lemon Yogurt, Sweetened with

**Lunch**

1 Cup Skim Milk

1 Cup Tossed Salad Mix

1 Tablespoon Fat Free French Salad Dressing

Chicken & White Bean Soup

2 Slices Reduced-Calorie Oatmeal Bran Bread

**Dinner**

1/2 Cup Cooked Quinoa

Bistro Beef Tenderloin

Roasted Baby Bok Choy

1 Cup Strawberries

# Calories and body reconstruction

The energy provided by food calories is needed for every function of the body, including healing, thought, physical activity, and growth. According to Medline Plus, "foods containing an equal number of calories and nutrients are ideal for a balanced diet". Proteins, carbohydrates, and fats are the building blocks of energy. After ingestion, carbohydrates are broken down into glucose, which provides raw energy that is either used immediately. Complex carbohydrates like whole grains, vegetables and fruits provide a balance of calories and nutrients, which is good for your overall heath. A healthy diet helps maintain an ideal body weight and prevent obesity. Empty calories, such as those derived from foods with little nutritional value can lead to weight gain. Eating foods with a balance of calories and nutrients can help provide the body with the fuel it needs to function while avoiding weight gain.

# Day 6 meal plan

**Breakfast**

1 Cup Skim Milk

1 Whole-Wheat English Muffin

1 Teaspoon Creamy Peanut Butter

1 Tablespoon Sugar-Free Jam

MORNING SNACK

1 Orange, medium

**Lunch**

1 Cup Skim Milk

1 Whole-Wheat Pita Bread, small

1 Cup Watermelon

**Dinner**

2/3 Cup Cooked Brown Rice

Green Salad with Asparagus & Peas.

1 Cup Cantaloupe Melon

# T-Shirt Dilemma

There's one white T-shirt in my black bag that I got from my brother for years, but I don't wear it, mainly because I think it's sort of represent who I used to be too much. It reads: "Eat Less you fat goat". Since it was my brother that gave it to me, I thought it was more of a joke and I don't take it too seriously. He had the shirts specifically made for me because he thought I needed to lose weight. However, the more I engage with the message of the shirt the more I consider what it means to eat less.  Over time I began to appreciate the message more, because it motivates me.

# American Dilemma

The average American now eats a ton of food that is roughly around 1,995 pounds per year. Between 1972s and 2001, Americans has increased its daily caloric intake by 20.5 percent. It's thus an experiential fact that majority of Americans, who consume about 3,500 calories daily need to reduce this number of calories. Americans today consume about 59 percent more meat than we did in the 1960s. We eat four times more yogurt, 20 times more corn sweetener, eight times more cheese, and 18 percent more wheat flour. These goods require more resources to produce and they emit more greenhouse gasses than their lower impact counterpart such as namely fresh vegetable and fruit. But as far as produce goes, Americans have only increased consumption modestly since the 1960s. Total fruit consumption had risen by a comparatively low 19 percent between 1960s and 2002, while total vegetable consumption has gone up 30 percent. One study concluded that if Americans reduced caloric intake to 2,500 calories per day, the carbon "food print" of the American diet would drop by 13 percent.

# DAY 7 meal plan

**Breakfast**

1 Cup Skim Milk

1 Plum

Taco

**SNACK**

1 Apple, small

**Lunch**

1 Veggie Burger

1 Whole-Wheat Roll

Bok Choy-Apple Slaw

1 Apricot

**Dinner**

1 Cup Skim Milk

1 Cup Tossed Salad Mix

1 Tablespoon Low Calorie Caesar Salad Dressing

Grilled Pork Tenderloin Marinated in Spicy Soy Sauce

1/2 Cup Cooked Brown Rice

# Benefits of eating less

Dietary choices that include less calorie intake are beneficial for our hormones. This is particularly applicable to eating less of fried and cholesterol foods that tend to impact the sexual and reproductive hormones. With lesser energy resources directed towards digesting food and removing toxins, the cells have more time to carry-out essential repair work. This means the skin can be protected against aging caused by free radicals. This also works towards faster regeneration of new, tighter tissues and slower aging of the skin. Thus, by eating less you have a greater chance towards looking younger and losing weight over time.

Eating lesser food means that your body is supplied with limited calorie intake. The body needs to carefully process every bit of food that you consume. The digestion is directed at maximizing nutrient absorption and minimal storage of unwanted calories as fat. Medical researchers across the world have repeatedly proven a direct relation between eating lesser and improving the brain's performance. This includes the cognitive abilities and overall IQ. In fact, limited dietary intake to sharpen the mind has been practiced in many cultures that existed thousands of years ago. It has been established that eating smaller portions and at regular intervals rather than having heavy meals is more likely to raise your ability to learn and memorize with ease. You might not realize this but a lot of diseases are the result of inflammations within the body. This means they are caused without an external cause like an infection. This happens when the body is unable to get rid of the toxins found in food. This kind of toxin retention is more likely to happen when we eat more.

# Using the information

Now that most of you understand how food function. Your next step is to use this information to improve your body physique. My hope is that you could benefits mentality as well as physically from everything that this information emphasizes. Often time people want to lose weight, but after a month they quit. You must be willing to go the extra mile, always tell yourself that you can do it. Nothing in life come easy, if you want something badly, set your goals and go after it. This meal plan will certainly help you as it has help me astronomically over the years.

# Conclusion

Thank you for choosing my book! I know that you already seen thousands of books on how to lose weight, but you have taken the chance to read mine. Thank you for the opportunity! And before you close this book I have one small request. When you turn over this page you will have the opportunity to share your thoughts about the book with your friends on Instagram, Facebook and twitter. If you think this information is worth it, please tell your friends. If it helps someone become more healthy and confident, they would be grateful to you. Now all you have to do is follow the 7-day meal plan and you will lose weight.

# About the author

Noel Johnson is a nutrition expert and health consultant. He received his degree in integrative and functional nutrition. He has pursued his passion helping people stay healthy and practice nutritional behavior to improve individual lifestyle. His aim is to help people lose weight by eating right, rather than committing to intense exercises and hard diet.

www.ingramcontent.com/pod-product-compliance
Lightning Source LLC
Chambersburg PA
CBHW071143280526
45787CB00003B/1384